HELP IS HOPE

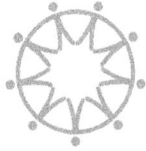

HELP IS HOPE

DEALING WITH CHRONIC ILLNESS

GINNY MASULLO

Turtle Lake Press
Fayetteville, Arkansas

ISBN-13: 978-0-615-47574-5
Library of Congress Control Number: 2012931022

Editor: Amy L. Wilson

Book Design & Cover Art: Susan Idlet & Dot Neely

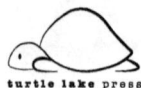

turtle lake press

1833 E. Applebury Drive, Fayetteville, Arkansas 72701
turtlelakepress.com

"Shared joy is a double joy; shared sorrow is half a sorrow."

—Swedish Proverb

"It'll matter who you touch and it matters what you give.

It'll matter if you try and makes a difference that you lived.

We're not here for very long. It's the only chance you've got.

You may be thinking that it is time to wait, but I am thinking that it's not."

—from the song "It'll Matter" by Nick Masullo

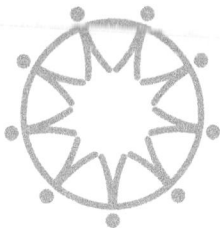

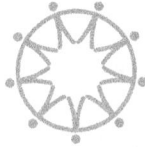

CONTENTS

HELP IS HOPE

INTRODUCTION

I WANTED TO RUN

My husband Nick and I had been married twenty-four years when he was diagnosed with primary progressive multiple sclerosis (PPMS). Nick, a singer songwriter, had just released his first CD of original songs. In his day job, he managed a natural foods coop. He was also a Special Olympics ice-skating coach and played hockey in his spare time.

The diagnosis explained his recent loss of balance, hearing loss, and increased fatigue. It also explained his significant loss of interest in our once robust sex life that had left me wondering about the fidelity of our relationship.

As a registered nurse, I had an all too clear picture of what might lie in store for Nick. I kept the scenarios I foresaw to myself because Nick expressed the verve and optimism that he could beat the devastating disease.

For the first couple of years—thanks to him being able to resign from his demanding full-time job and draw disability—Nick could administer most of his care himself. He tried fifty-three different treatment modalities. One of these involved bee stings for nine months several times a week, which I administered. Others, recommended by his neurologist, included injections for the remitting type of MS, as well as chemotherapy.

In those first years, Nick prided himself on his self-care. This entailed taking as much as an hour just to get dressed. For each loss, which came monthly, he adapted. He had an incredible store of determination.

When he couldn't write with his right hand anymore, he learned to write with his left. He continued to compose songs. As playing the guitar became more difficult, he devised ways to make his guitar picks stay in his unreliable hands. When he could still drive his handicapped van, he drove himself to the farmers market and played for listeners on our town square. He felt strongly that it was important for him to be out in the world, no matter that he was now handicapped. Nick saw the bigger picture; he was one person but representing many like himself. By the time he could no longer walk, a friend dubbed him *"the cheerful cripple."*

With me he showed another side, talking about suicide and asking me if I would perform euthanasia for him. By this time, so much paralysis had taken over his body that his only option for unassisted suicide would be to choose not eating or drinking.

Before being faced with the actual situation of helping a loved one literally cross over, I had thought that assisting someone with suicide would be something I could do. When it came down to it, however, I realized I couldn't. I shared this revelation with Nick, adding that if he decided to choose the option of not eating or drinking, I would be supportive. From the time those conversations began until his death, Nick led a productive and creative life despite the continual assaults on his body. He produced three more CDs of original songs and two books of essays. And, he continued to ask me about euthanasia.

At the time of his diagnosis, our oldest son was completing his master's degree and our sixteen-year-old son was college-bound. I worked part-time as a nurse in a university clinic. Fortunately, I was able to increase my hours in order to obtain insurance benefits for the family.

Just before the diagnosis, Nick had begun pursuing his music as never before. Meanwhile, I had been mining my creative urges in writing. I had a weekly poetry column in the local paper, and through classes and mentors, I'd begun to pursue fiction writing and poetry. However, as Nick's care became more demanding, all of my creative pursuits had to go. His needs became the focus of my world.

When he could no longer control his bowels, a morning program was required to prevent accidents. For me, this eventually meant arising at 4 a.m. to get Nick showered, dressed and in his electric wheelchair so that he could lead his day at home. For a few months, he could prepare his own food from his chair. When he could no longer do that, he could get food I prepared for him from the counter or fridge. Eventually, he could no longer feed himself or drink water without assistance. Often, I would come home on my lunch hour to help him eat and transfer him back to bed for a much needed rest.

I wanted to run. *"How can I possibly keep up this schedule,"* I cried to my art therapist. *"You need help,"* she said flatly. Nick agreed, somewhat reluctantly. The idea of other people coming to his house was anathema to a man who did not like more than the occasional visitor in our home in even the best of times.

We began the search for a paid morning aide. We interviewed both a private agency and interviewed individuals from a list that the local Schmieding Center on Aging provided. We tried three different individuals before we found the appropriate fit with Jack, who stayed for over three years until Nick's death.

We could not afford Jack for more than two to three hours a day, four days a week. The lunch and afternoon transfer remained along with the late afternoon transfer, dinner, and the care required in the evening for bed among a multitude of other things, such as shopping, typing for Nick, bill paying, and just plain human interaction during the day.

My therapist encouraged me to call together a group of friends to brainstorm about ways to create more help for the mounting tasks required to keep Nick at home. The group gathered monthly for over two years. From their support and ideas, a circle of care grew over time, a circle that filled many of the needs. Before that circle, those tasks were in my hands. I'd felt consistently overwhelmed and inadequate and not a little angry with our lot in life.

At first, Nick voiced resistance to the idea of a revolving door of volunteers. However, once he became directly involved by making contacts for help himself, he experienced the kindnesses of those who wanted to help, and he became enthusiastic. Now, instead of a tired, overwhelmed wife assisting him with various tasks, an interesting assortment of fresh and ready hands came to his aid.

Nick and I together made a list of things that needed doing on a regular basis. When we asked for help, it would be for a specific task at a specific time, with the goal being no more than an hour at a time for most helpers. A schedule was made and volunteers were asked to find their own replacements from the list of substitutes we made.

We did a lot of asking for help. I admit that the asking never got easy, but it did get less uncomfortable as time went on. People I had expected to become involved because of a long friendship did not necessarily step up. This felt bewildering at first, but Nick and I came to understand that people do what they can when they can for all manner of reasons. We learned that expectations were not appropriate and that help often came from astonishing corners. For example, musicians collaborated with Nick on his songs when he could no longer play or sing but could compose. They produced albums and helped put together fund-raising and awareness-raising events and concerts.

Eventually, when swallowing became difficult and he stated he would not want any intervention, Nick was placed on hospice. That added another circle within the wheel, a circle that lasted two years.

Even with all the many circles in our wheel of help, the journey felt arduous and complicated. Having so many people in our lives, sometimes six or seven daily, felt both joyful and challenging. I felt embarrassed about things like taking a nap on Saturday afternoon while someone else helped Nick. Scheduling did not always go as designed. I might have to cancel a plan I'd made if a helper cancelled.

The gains, however, far exceeded the frustrations. Over time, I began to feel like I could breathe again. I took a watercolor class and found some time to write poetry. Nick and I spent time together that felt more like the husband and wife relationship we had felt before the ravages of MS. I stopped raging against fate and accepted our circumstances with a gratitude for the goodness that came mixed with the pain.

If I could have chosen, I would not have elected the lives to which MS led Nick and me. In the beginning, Nick truly thought he could beat the disease, but that was not how things turned out. Even so, while MS wrecked his body, it did not destroy him as a person. As he said in his essay *Being Healed*, "It might be possible to be healed with MS even if I might not be healed from MS." (See page 45.)

It's true enough, and part of that healing came from the circle of care that surrounded him. I too benefited from that circle of caring individuals. At the end of the day, I was not broken as many full-time caregivers often are. That is not to say Nick and I both didn't struggle with the demons of resentment and bitterness from time to time. However, that is to say help is a soothing salve to those inevitable feelings that come with the losses and grief of chronic illness.

This manual and the essays that follow are framed with the wish that others may find similar hope for their own crisis of need.

CHAPTER 1

HELP IS OXYGEN

If chronic illness visits your house, you will need help. Help is oxygen. One's whole world is rocked. Finances and physical energy are sapped. Depression often sets in for the one with the problem and those closest to them.

I learned that fact the hard way when my 50-year-old husband of 25 years went from a highly active man playing ice hockey to a quadriplegic over a two-year period. For several more years he required help with every activity of daily living, from taking a sip of water to getting dressed to toileting to moving his limbs.

With the help of my therapist and friends, we organized a circle of help that eventually grew to 70 volunteer slots a month and lasted for more than three years. For his morning program, we hired an aide. Nick was able to stay at home until he passed away.

After Nick died, several people approached me about setting up similar care circles. That's when I realized the need for a handbook that would guide others in the process. I solicited the assistance of several women. We brainstormed about the presentation and mechanics, which led to the no-frills approach of this handbook.

While we met periodically to create this booklet, a woman some of us knew struggled with cancer. She lived alone and had resided in Fayetteville only a short time. Could a care circle or helping wheel work for her like it had for my husband, who had resided in our town for years and who knew hundreds of people? The model was put to the test, and in a short time, a helping wheel started rolling for her. While she did not have as much help as Nick, her wheel of help provided significant assistance and hope not only for her but also for her mother, her primary caregiver. The basic information here is meant to get you on your way to receiving help, as well as to highlight the most important elements on which to concentrate when devastating illness hits.

CHAPTER 2

HELP IS HOPE - GETTING STARTED

Envision a system of circles at the center of which is the person to be helped. Around him or her is a small circle of people who oversee and monitor the helping process, one or more of whom coordinate the help. Surrounding them are intersecting circles of friends, family members, organizations, and others who agree to perform specific tasks for the person being helped. Help is hope. To the persons who need the help and are already overwhelmed, this initial set-up may sound impossible. It is not. Read on to learn the concrete steps to take.

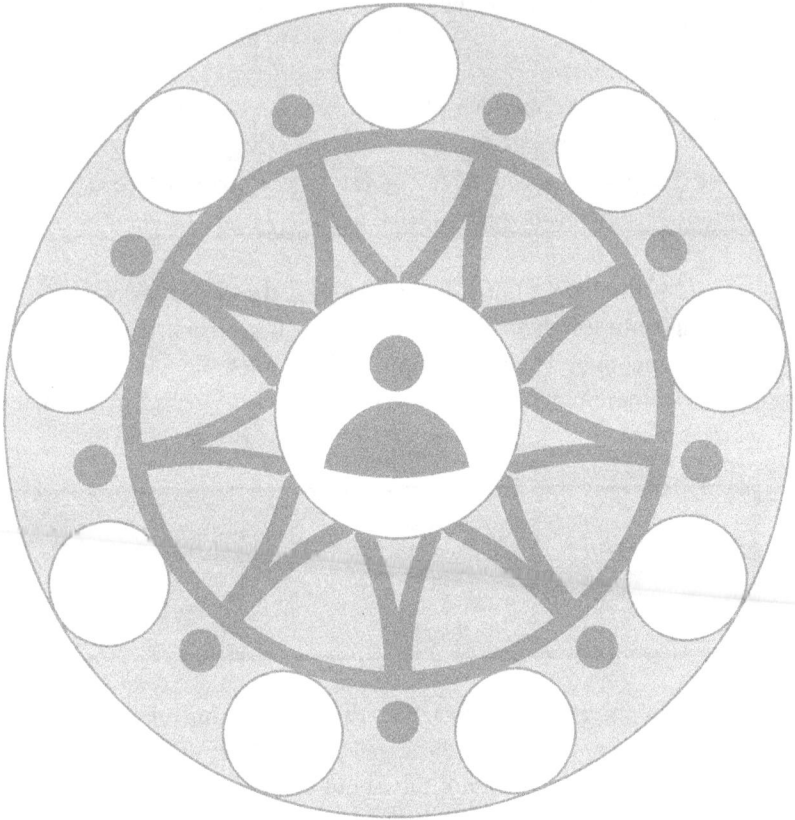

STEP 1
ESTABLISHING THE CORE GROUP

The core group oversees the care process. The person or family needing help is asked for names of people who might help with organizing the assistance. This might consist of 3 to 6 people. One or two of the core group agree to coordinate the help.

List the names and contact information of possible core group members. Then, contact the possible core group members to ask them if they would be willing to meet routinely to oversee the process of getting help for the person.

SAMPLE CONTACT DIALOGUE

"We are setting up a round-robin of care and a support group for_____. We need a core group that will initiate the round-robin and continue to oversee the process. We will meet one to two times a month to assess needs and establish a wheel of helpers to meet those needs. Would you be willing to be part of that group? Please know that your saying 'yes' does not mean 'yes' forever, just for now. Nor does it mean you will necessarily do any of the tasks other than organizational work."

If they are willing, ask for several times that would be a good meeting time for them. Tell them you will get back with them about the first meeting. Then, set a time and place for the first meeting. This may take some juggling until you can find what works for the majority of members.

DATE/TIME	
PLACE	

Be aware of the fact that the membership of the group may change over time. The first three meetings will occur in a short time and thereafter, monthly or bimonthly should work.

CORE GROUP

POSSIBLE CORE MEMBER	CONTACT INFORMATION

STEP 2
ORGANIZING THE FIRST MEETING

At the first meeting, decide these things:

1. Who will be the coordinator(s) of help for the person requiring assistance? The coordinators need to know that they are just that. They will not necessarily be performing tasks or substituting, although they may do all three. However, the point is to spread out the care rather than allowing many tasks to fall to a few.

2. Of the coordinators, determine who will meet with the person needing help to obtain information about possible helpers and about the tasks that need to be done. Begin a list at this meeting of people that the core members think might participate. Offer that list to the person needing care as a starting point for them. Be sure to brainstorm about specific organizations such as home health agencies, hospice, and faith-based groups.

3. Plan generally how the core group will disseminate information about who needs help and what needs to be done. (This planning may not be completed until after obtaining specific information from the person needing help.) At the end of each meeting, always set a time and place for the next meeting.

DATE/TIME	
PLACE	

COORDINATORS	CONTACT INFORMATION

POSSIBLE HELPERS	CONTACT INFORMATION

See Appendix for Additional List Templates.

STEP 3
MEETING WITH THE PERSON NEEDING CARE

The coordinators meet with the person needing care to ask for possible sources of help and list or lists of tasks that need to be done.

POSSIBLE SOURCES OF HELP

List any sources of help, including clubs, organizations, family members, friends, and faith-based groups. With clubs, include groups like gardening club, bridge club, or Rotary Club. With organizations, include health care providers such as home health, private care providers, and hospice if appropriate. See the "Resources" section for more about health care providers and disease-specific organizations.

Remember that people want to help if they can. You will get some "no" answers and you will get some "yes" answers. Having core group members do the initial asking assists those in need in getting over the tremendous hurdle of asking for help.

YOUR PLACE OF WORK

Unfortunately, despite great strides that have been made in the workplace to prevent discrimination against people who are ill or are caring for an ill family member, you must consider how to proceed in regard to the consequences of telling or not telling. The potential for discrimination is hard to predict and may differ according to the illness, job, status in the workplace, and the nature of your relationships at work. Ultimately, some measure of disclosure is likely to be necessary. Asking coworkers to be part of your helping wheel could have varying effects, so think carefully before you *do* include coworkers.

Whatever your degree of disclosure, remember to "walk tall" and know your legal rights. Continue to assure your workplace that you want to perform well at work *and* provide the care that your loved one needs. Do not buy into the all too prevalent attitude that, just because illness is in your house, you are somehow less of a person or less of a good employee.

HUMAN RESOURCES DEPARTMENT AS A RESOURCE

Go to your Human Resources Department (HRD) to determine what other types of assistance are available through your institution. There may be free or low-cost counseling or an employee-run fund to help with personal crisis.

FAMILY AND MEDICAL LEAVE ACT

Determine whether you are covered by the Family and Medical Leave Act, signed by President Clinton in 1993. Provisions in the act guarantee certain workers up to 12 weeks of unpaid, job-protected medical leave when the employee is unable to work because of a serious health condition or needs to care for an immediate family member (spouse, child, or parent) with a serious health condition.

ORGANIZATIONS

NAME OF ORGANIZATION	CONTACT INFORMATION

REGULAR HELPERS

NAME	CONTACT INFORMATION

SUBSTITUTE HELPERS

NAME	CONTACT INFORMATION

STEP 4
DETERMINING THE TASKS

BE SPECIFIC

The more specific the time and task the easier it is for the helper to commit. Knowing there is a beginning and ending time makes it easier for people to include another commitment in their busy lives. Being clear about what is needed during that time is also useful to the people who are being asked to help. While it may seem difficult at first, in the long run this specificity helps everyone. Tasks get done and people who want to help feel they have accomplished their assignment.

LIST TASKS NEEDED

Group tasks into categories such as: Childcare. Companionship. Doctor's appointments. Medications. Meals. Personal care. Respite care. Shopping. Skilled nursing. Transfers from bed to chair. Typing.

Define what tasks or chores would be easiest to ask others to do, which tasks the person or their partner must do and which tasks, if any, can be paid for. Consider that there is more than one person who needs assistance. The person with the health crisis is the most obvious. The primary caregiver is in need as well, but may be so accustomed to carrying several loads that they find it difficult to list even one task that would lessen their load, such as a night away from home or a meal carried in.

Some tasks are small and some require skill and/or great patience. Everyone has some special ability that can be utilized. One person might be quite comfortable with hands-on care while another might be best at helping with shopping or childcare or computer work. Throw away your expectations. Someone you might expect to do hands-on care might be more comfortable with offering shopping or being a substitute.

TASKS

The energy created by even a small group of people
sharing a load is astounding.

TASK	TIMEFRAME	COMMENTS

STEP 5
HOLDING SECOND CORE GROUP MEETING

PREPARATION

1. Make copies of tasks and potential volunteers' contact information.
2. Using an empty calendar with no dates, only days, assign tasks and times to calendar. While there are electronic methods for doing this, filling in by hand may be just as easy and accessible to everyone.
3. Make copies.

SECOND MEETING OF CORE GROUP

1. Hand out copies.
2. Prioritize which tasks need to be done sooner.
3. Initial by potential volunteers who will contact whom and for what job.
4. Know that there may be some overlap that will need to be ironed out.
5. Set a time frame for accomplishing the first round of contacts.

Personal contacts initially are better than group e-mail, but each situation merits a different mode of communication. Group e-mails should definitely be made, once a volunteer list has been established.

SAMPLE CONTACT DIALOGUE
"We are setting up round-robin care for _____. *Would you be willing to help? Here are the tasks and times that these things need to be done."* If they say they cannot commit to a regular time, ask if they would be willing to be placed on a back-up list. Explain: *"The back-up list is used when regulars need a substitute or when new needs arise. Would you be willing to be on that list?"*

Organize the scheduling of tasks as people volunteer to help. Fill in the calendar with the acknowledged commitments. These calendars, along with the two lists of regulars and substitutes, are distributed to everyone involved. Hard copies are left in the home of the people being served.

METHODS FOR SCHEDULING

There are several options here, but the efficacy of these methods depends upon each member being computer literate enough to use the site. If the electronic method seems the best, training could be provided. One such internet site is called lotsahelpinghands.com at which information about a particular person may be listed. People may sign up and be accepted to volunteer on behalf of the person. The benefit of the site is that the calendar is interactive and immediately shows which tasks are covered and which are not. The downside to the site is that it takes computer-savvy to set up the site and administer it. Also, tasks can only be listed for particular times and days – there is no allowance for signing up for tasks which can be done anytime.

Another method of creating a task schedule is to post a large calendar at the person's home on which people may sign up for future tasks when there.

Regardless of the method, everyone involved has a list of the other helpers. When a helper cannot keep his/her scheduled time, he/she finds a replacement and then informs the person being helped of this change.

COMMUNICATION MODES

Based on my experience, e-mails and phone calls proved to be the best methods of communication across all age groups and seemed to be much more effective than electronic calendars.

YOUR PRIVACY

The reality of so many people coming into your home at all hours may seem distasteful and at times you may long for more privacy, but think about the alternatives, such as institutionalization of your loved one. The caregiver who is being relieved needs to know he/she does not need to entertain or host everyone who comes to the house. People who are helping need to realize this as well.

Over time, the schedule can be changed if there is the unlikely situation of too much help. Should a helper not be a good fit, this can be discussed by the core group and handled appropriately.

CORE GROUP MEETINGS

The core group meets on a regular basis to strategize about changing needs and to evaluate how the entire program is working or not working. A designated facilitator keeps the meeting focused by opening the meeting with the agenda. Once care is ongoing, one to two times a month should be adequate. At the meeting these areas are addressed:

1. A report from the primary caregiver and the person receiving help may include any new needs or concerns, any gaps in care, what is working, and what is not working.
2. Recruitment of other volunteers.
3. Any needed changes for core members.
4. Other agenda items should be added at the beginning of the meeting.

Try to keep the meeting to one to two hours at most. Knowing you need to wrap things up in a set amount of time helps people stay focused. Acknowledge at each meeting that it will be the facilitator's job to keep the focus on the agenda items.

The meetings may need to include the actual person in need and/or the significant other of that person. Every situation is different and ever-changing. Whatever the circumstances, the person being helped needs to feel a major level of input into the process.

CHAPTER 3

ASKING FOR HELP

Yes, all this involves coordination and an initial output of energy. The primary caregiver or the person in need might be tempted to say, "Oh, it is easier to just do the tasks myself." Not wanting to accept help is the main pitfall of caregivers and those in need, warns the Caregiver Action Network.

Asking for help is more a sign of strength than weakness. It means that a plan of action is in place. Still, there is a fine line between expectation and hope. Hope is good. Expectation is not. You will get a "yes" answer sometimes and a "no" answer other times. Do not take the "no" responses personally. Just move down your list of potential helpers. Ask with a matter-of-fact tone. Know that you may never get over the feeling of being an imposition. Know and believe that people *do* want to help. By asking and providing them with a specific task, you are helping them feel they can offer a measure of service in what may otherwise feel like an untenable situation.

CHAPTER 4

APPLYING FOR SOCIAL SECURITY DISABILITY

If someone is ill and/or disabled, whether it seems temporary or not, you may want to consider filing for Social Security Disability sooner rather than later. There are a number of reasons for this.

If a person is unable to work and decides to live off her savings until her health improves, she may go broke before her health improves. Not only would her savings be depleted, but the fact that she has not been working could decrease the chance of qualifying. In order to satisfy the definition of disability used by Social Security, a person's disability or impairment must meet or equal the level of severity described in the Social Security listing book.

Disability claims can take a very long time to process. This isn't true in all cases, but it is in most. Unfortunately, many claimants for disability benefits have experienced severe problems and hardship simply because they had no idea how long the process would take, and only realized when it was too late that they should have filed an application much sooner. Once on Social Security Disability, there is often a waiting period to receive Medicare benefits. Sometimes there are exceptions to the latter statement. Consult with a lawyer who specializes in this area and check out ssa.gov/disability.

RESOURCES

AREA AGENCIES ON AGING

There are Area Agencies on Aging in each state throughout the United States. They can usually answer basic information on local available resources for caregivers and people 65 and older. If you are not 65 or older, they may well be a good starting place anyway.

Also, a local Department of Human Services may have an Office on Aging or programs to assist people with disabilities under age 65. In addition, many national organizations have local affiliates for particular diseases, such as the American Parkinson's Disease Association (APDA) and Alzheimer's Association. These groups often offer emotional support and education close to home.

MEDICARE

Medicare is a health insurance program into which workers pay. It is for seniors 65 years and older or those receiving Social Security Disability. Medicare does not pay for personal care (also known as "custodial care" or "non-medical care"). Medicare will pay for a very limited number of days of skilled nursing (also referred to as "nursing home care"). Medicare will also pay for some home health care, provided it is medical in nature. (See the section on applying for disability.)

MEDICAID

Medicaid is a state-specific insurance program for low-income individuals with limited financial assets. Medicaid, being state run, has different benefits in each state. Generally speaking, Medicaid pays for nursing home care through waiver programs, home care, personal care, and assisted living. To avoid confusion, it is worth noting that Medicaid is referred to by different names in different states. Medicaid is **not** Medicare and is administered at the county level. To apply for Medicaid, visit your local Social Services office.

HOME HEALTH

Home health care simply means providing medically-related services to patients in a home setting rather than in a medical facility. Home health care may include skilled nursing in addition to speech, occupational, and physical therapy. Paid out of pocket, it can be expensive. However, do not assume that these services cost too much. Ask for an evaluation either by calling your doctor and asking for a referral or calling the agency who will ask the doctor for a referral. The agency should do a free evaluation and Medicare often covers such services when certain criteria are met. Private health insurance often does too.

IN HOME CARE

As a general rule, "in home" services typically provide help with day-to-day tasks such as cooking, cleaning, and shopping. Usually, there is a cost involved. However, people may qualify for help from agencies such as Area Agency for the Aging. Again, it's always best to ask for an evaluation. Don't assume you can't get or afford help.

HOSPICE

Most people think hospice means your loved one has a diagnosis of less than six months to live, and with some hospice situations, a year. While that is technically true, some people receive hospice or "palliative" services for much longer. Palliative means comfort measures rather than curative measures.

A good rule of thumb is to call hospice sooner rather than later. Hospice care can dramatically improve the quality of one's life. Hospice services can include doctors, nurses, physical therapy, social workers, chaplains, and volunteers. Hospice workers are experts in pain control and provide an on call nurse 24/7 to consult when problems arise.

Anyone can inquire about hospice services. Hospice staff will contact your physician to determine if a referral to hospice is appropriate. Another way to inquire about hospice is to talk with your physician. He/she can make a referral to hospice. Hospice can begin as soon as a referral is made by the person's doctor. Hospice is not a free service unless you are on Medicare. However, an evaluation should be requested. Hospice will help explore options. Visit www.nhpco.org, the website for National Hospice and Palliative Care Organization, for more information.

PALLIATIVE CARE

Palliative care focuses on relief from symptoms, pain, and the stress of serious illness—whatever the diagnosis. The goal is to improve quality of life for both the patient and the family.

Palliative care is provided by a team of doctors, nurses, and other specialists who work together with a patient's other doctors to provide an extra layer of support. It is appropriate at any age and at any stage in a serious illness and can be provided along with curative treatment. (In hospice care, palliative care is integral, but curative treatments are no longer considered viable.) For more information, visit www.getpalliativecare.org.

DISEASE-SPECIFIC ORGANIZATIONS

Check the internet for an extensive list of disease-specific organizations or call the Family Caregiver Alliance® at (415) 434-3388 or (800) 445-8106. You may also e-mail the Family Care Alliance at info@caregiver.org or visit their website (caregiver.org).

OTHER ORGANIZATIONS

- Well Spouse (wellspouse.org) provides support for spouses.
- Caregivers Resources (usa.gov/Citizen/Topics/Health.shtml) helps you locate a nursing home, assisted living, or hospice; check your eligibility for benefits; get resources for long-distance caregiving; review legal issues; and find support for caregivers.
- Caregiver Action Network (caregiveraction.org) is a non-profit organization (formerly the National Family Caregivers Association) that provides free education, peer support, and resources to family members who are caring for loved ones with chronic conditions, disabilities, disease, or the frailties of old age.

- Caring Bridge (www.caringbridge.org) offers free personalized websites to people facing a serious medical condition or hospitalization, undergoing medical treatment and/or recovering from a significant accident, illness, injury, or procedure. The service allows family members and friends to receive consistent information via a single website, and eliminates the need to place and receive numerous telephone calls.
- Lotsahelpinghands (info@lotsahelpinghands.com) will assist you in the creation of a free private online community to organize support for caregivers, friends, and colleagues. Their vision is "a world where everyone can give and receive help through the power of community."

FURTHER READING

While there are many good books on caregiving, *Passages in Caregiving* by Gail Sheehy (William Morrow, 2010) provides a wealth of helpful information and additional resources.

ESSAYS

GINNY SPEAKS

AFTER THE HOLIDAYS

Anyone can stop a man's life, but no one his death;
a thousand doors open on to it.
Seneca

Before dawn on a December morning in 2007, Jack, our morning aide called in sick. This meant that Nick would need to wake up three hours earlier than usual so that I could perform his morning program before I left the house at 7:30.

I would feed him, give him his meds, place a suppository, get him out of bed into his rolling shower chair, perform his bowel program, shower him, return him to bed where I would dress him, and finally transfer him to his power chair. He would spend the rest of the morning listening to the radio, unable to even drink water, until a volunteer came at noon to feed him lunch and transfer him back to bed for an afternoon rest.

As I turned off the water of the shower wand and patted his hair dry with a towel, he said, "I think, after Christmas, I'll stop eating or drinking." I felt like I had inhaled the dry dust of a leaf. I kept drying his hair, speechless, confused, and not a little angry that he would bring up such a serious topic when we, at least I, felt crunched for time.

Two years before, in 2005, Nick had talked so much about euthanasia that we called the Death with Dignity National Center in Oregon. We were able to engage in a phone conference. We found out that since I was unwilling to help Nick, by my own hands, pass out of this world, the only option open to him was to decide to not eat or drink. "Pretty grim," he said when we hung up. When the promised written information arrived from the organization, I placed it in a drawer, thinking I would pull it out if Nick asked for it. He didn't.

Instead he continued to compose original songs, record CDs, and even perform in public with the help of fellow musicians. He worked constantly in his head on two eventual books of essays.

When swallowing became increasingly difficult and Nick expressed clearly that he did not want any heroic measures such as resuscitation, the calling of 911, or even the Heimlich maneuver should he choke, we called our local hospice.

When to my surprise they did admit him to their home visit program, Nick asked me, "So when are they going to help me die?"

The wife in me kept quiet with my incredulity. When I had been a hospice nurse over eight years before, did Nick think I ran around the rural homes of the Ozarks like Dr. Kevorkian, helping people end their lives? The nurse in me explained to him the principles of hospice care. "They are not in the business of euthanasia. In fact, their goal is to increase the quality of your life knowing the end of it may be near."

Indeed, hospice did improve both of our lives. For me, hospice lifted a considerable weight from my shoulders. It meant I had someone else with whom I could discuss wound care or call upon to change his leaking urinary catheter when my leaving work would create problems. It meant I could be more of a companion than a nurse, at least some of the time. Nick's quality of life improved as well. The fact is that despite my own training, our hospice nurses had tricks that neither our doctor nor I had thought of. For instance, the glycerin spray they provided helped Nick to swallow with a little more ease. He coughed and choked less when eating. By contrast, the throat specialist had only offered a feeding tube. Hospice provided creative and practical ways to more comfortably manage issues that could not be fixed.

When Nick informed me in the shower on that gray December morning in 2007 that "after the holidays he would stop eating or drinking," he had been on hospice much longer than most hospice patients. I felt stressed to not miss work. My working, after all, made health coverage for our family possible. Work was essential to maintaining the delicate balance of our lives in the face of Nick's illness. I also knew that asking too many questions often backfired. Nick would clam up. I now regret not trying to explore his feelings right then and there.

When I arrived at work, a university medical clinic, the day was slow. I spent my lunch hour crying in the bathroom. I washed my face and called Nick. He answered with his hands-free device (supplied by the state of Arkansas). He sounded upbeat and his helper, Karen, laughed in the background. It felt as if he had never dropped the bomb "after the holidays."

That night in our dining room, as I fed him overdone ravioli, the silence between us felt thick. I wavered. If he didn't bring up "after the holidays," should I? I didn't, nor did he.

Christmas came. We celebrated with friends and family. Carolers visited our home on Christmas Eve. I made potato latkes for Nick at his request. I look back at photos of that Christmas. Nick looks ashen and gaunt but wears a Santa hat. He holds his friend Kelly's hand and they both laugh, looking into each other's eyes.

Nick did not speak again of not eating or drinking until the following September. Instead, almost weekly he would ask me if I could end his life. I'd remind him that I could not, would not. Or, he'd ask, "Do you think God would punish me if I ended my life?" I returned the question with questions. "Do you?" Since he had been raised Catholic, he said that he might be held accountable. However, when I asked him if he thought I might be punished if I overdosed him at his request, he stated an emphatic "no!"

One of my regrets is that when he would raise these questions, I did not find a way to more fully meet him in his anguish. Was I too focused and stressed from working fulltime and care giving? Did I focus too much on strategizing on the many everyday needs? I still grapple with that concern. I want to learn how to just sit with another in the inevitable pain of living.

Infections for Nick became more frequent. Pain increased and Nick, who for 25 years had not used any caffeine or alcohol, let alone drugs, began to take prescription pain meds. On Friday, September 5, 2008, Nick called me at work on his voice-activated phone. "Should I take these antibiotics?"

He'd been struggling with a respiratory illness that the hospice nurse decided might be pneumonia. At that time, our hospice considered antibiotics a gray area. Were antibiotics considered curative or palliative?

In this case, they offered antibiotics to Nick as a comfort measure. I thought of his recent request to help him out of his misery. My detached nurse persona kicked in (I was at work, after all). I replied, "They say that pneumonia is the old man's friend." Immediately, I wanted to retract that statement and said, "Nick, I can't talk about this over the phone. Let's talk about it when I get home. Order the antibiotics and then you can decide."

I called a friend and asked her to meet me at home later that evening. As it turned out, Nick's best friend, Barbara, would be coming to help Nick up before I arrived home. I thought perhaps the four of us could discuss the antibiotics question with him as a group. While it was an intimate decision, I felt great need for witnesses and help.

I told my boss about the call. "This is what I have to deal with." For the first time in the five years of Nick's steady decline, she suggested I consider taking family leave. I replied, "This could go on for a long time. I might need it later more than now."

When I arrived home, Nick sat in his power chair and Barbara sat on our red couch. On the table, five letters were laid out. Nick had composed the letters weeks before and dictated them to his friend, Jeanie, who volunteered her time to enter his work into the computer. There was a personal letter to me, a letter to each of our sons, a letter to be read at his memorial, and the following letter.

FOR MY BEDSIDE

Dear Friends,

I've had enough. Actually, more than enough. I will not be eating or drinking. We have consulted with the Death with Dignity folks in Oregon, and they say that is my best option. I have tried to live with dignity and even a little grace, and I will try to live that way up to the end. Thank you for making my life worth living.

Love, Nick

Given the course of events, his 2007 pre-holiday statement, infections, pain, and drugs, and his repeated plea for euthanasia, I should not have been surprised. Yet his decision felt like an unwelcome specter turned real.

"What about the CD release concert you have planned for October?" I asked him.

"Let it be my memorial," he replied calmly.

Later, after Nick's death, I checked dates in the computer. At the same time that he dictated his letters, he also planned life, working on essays, ordering backup equipment in case controls broke in the future, and planning his CD and book release event in October.

The night of Nick's announcement of his decision, unbelievably, he suggested that we watch a movie, *The Italian Job*, with friends. My mind reeled. I did not call family immediately, thinking that one, Nick might change his mind, and two if not, then the ordeal would unfold over several days if not weeks. I also thought he and I would have time to talk.

Little did I imagine as I tossed and turned, sleepless through the night, that Nick would slip into a coma the very next day and cease breathing only hours later.

While I imagine a sudden unexpected death of a loved one, like an accident, to be more difficult than Nick's passing, I felt cheated. I had been so busy going through his Saturday morning routine, calling hospice, calling Nick's sisters and our sons, the regret of not just sitting with Nick in his sorrow remains to this day.

Fortunately, that regret is not all I have to dwell upon as I recall Nick's passing. Once he slipped into unconsciousness, I made more phone calls to friends and family. At the time of his last breath, friends surrounded his bed, playing music, touching him with love and concern, moving in and out of his room. I lay with him and held the phone to his ear as his sisters and our sons, who were en route, spoke to the place in Nick that I believe could still hear. Part of me wanted everyone to leave. Another part welled with gratitude for the cushion they created.

Nick's deathbed felt like a ferryboat. All of us were gathered to send him off on his journey to the other side.

THE BURIED HEART

Where does one go from a world of insanity?
Somewhere on the other side of despair.
T.S. Eliot

With primary progressive multiple sclerosis (PPMS) taking something from Nick almost every month, if not every week, I began to imagine that the onslaught might be a little like being in combat. Loss after loss. No time to process, just cope and put one foot in front of the other, do what needs to be done. Adapt. Bury your aching heart.

But whether it is war or disease, grief eventually finds its way into the psyche in the form of despair and sorrow.

Early on in Nick's struggle with PPMS I read a book, *Mainstay: For the Well Spouse of the Chronically Ill* by Maggie Strong. As wife and caregiver to her husband who had multiple sclerosis, her account of that experience pulled no punches about the stress of being a well spouse. She quoted a woman who said she tried to work her way around the wheel of emotions each day. It felt reassuring that this emotional lability might be more of a norm than an inadequacy on my part. I could go from crying inconsolably in the shower to laughing with a friend at work. I often felt terrified that when the despair or anger hit I would stay there and never get out.

Our culture primarily tells us to keep the stiff upper lip. If there is sorrow or loss, we need to be over it in a couple of weeks. If we are not, we are labeled pathological and likely offered medication. (Sometimes medication is a lifesaver.) I felt blue, defeated, and wrapped in the murky cloak of a low-grade depression. I criticized myself for my negative feelings. After all, I could still walk, bathe myself, and go to the bathroom without assistance. Yet despite the helping hands of family and friends, I sometimes felt remarkably lonely and isolated.

In Peter McWilliam's *You Can't Afford the Luxury of a Negative Thought*, I read the chapter on "Accentuate the Positive." In that section he included information on grieving. He wrote, "I include this information on grieving in this chapter on accentuating the positive because mourning is a positive human trait. It allows us the flexibility to adapt to change. It is not negative to feel pain and anger at loss. The negativity enters when the process of healing–which is in fact a gift–is denied."

What a relief it felt to read those words, to see that the sometimes overwhelming anger and pain could be a positive force. I found that if I let myself feel those emotions then the energy would move. Instead of feeling weighted down I would feel lighter, emptied. I did try to let those feelings find their honorable place in a private setting; I tried to be careful with whom I chose to share the darker emotions. This is not to say that the anger or pain didn't sometimes come out in a way that might be hurtful to Nick or someone else close. I hated it when that happened and had to learn to forgive myself.

I learned that the three stages of grief were by no means linear. They were a spinning circle of Shock/ Denial, Anger/ Depression, Understanding/ Acceptance, and then back again.

Life becomes loss any way you look at it, and illness has a way of reminding us of our common fragility and impermanence. I saw that in allowing the inevitable pain and sorrow to find its rightful place in the light, my buried heart started to open up to all the good that also manifested. I built an underlying foundation of acceptance that I could return to over and over.

I was helped to do this by another book, Miriam Greenspan's *Healing Through The Dark Emotions*.

Greenspan asks how can our children have faith in an adult world that cannot name despair in relation to the world. What kind of faith in life are we teaching them, that so closely resembles denial?

So I came to know that despair felt painful but it was not as disabling as I feared. The trick became how to be with others and be in such pain. I grapple still with this one. In my case, sharing my sense of grief and loss with Nick only added to his burden. The man who once gave me counsel and solace could not be those things to me.

How did I find the friend that could give such witness? I think I became that friend but with the help of counseling, the helping wheel, journaling, and process art. I went into the ravine alone and dug up my heart. Not all the time but some of the time, at least, I came to understand the words of the Greek playwright Aeschylus in *Agamemnon*:

He who learns must suffer.
And even in our sleep, pain that cannot forget falls drop by drop
upon the heart, and in our own despair, against our will,
comes wisdom through the awful grace of God.

We can only hope that the inevitable suffering of life will not be squandered, that it will make us wiser, more compassionate, more connected to the wheel of life and death.

NICK SPEAKS

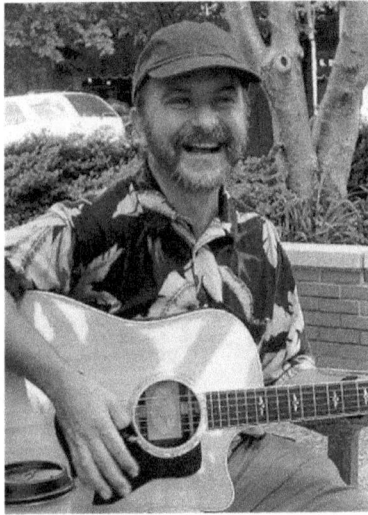

NICK MASULLO, 1952-2008

The following essays are excerpted and reprinted with permission from *Being Healed* by Nick Masullo, a collection published in 2008.

BEING HEALED

Perhaps I can be healed and still have MS. When I was first diagnosed, I was obsessed with quickly finding a cure. I read 30 books that had a positive slant on my condition and healing. I certainly wasn't going to be one of those people who ended up in a wheelchair. I had friends with MS who had become skeptical about finding a cure. I would show them.

I have now tried 40 different treatment modalities from the conventional to the experimental. I've tried daily self-injections of amino acids. I've tried alternative therapies of all kinds. I have been locked in a pressurized oxygen chamber daily for a month. I have been stung by 1,700 bees. I tried four months of chemotherapy. I have approached each of these modalities with hope and optimism.

I worked for 30 years distributing organic and natural foods and supplements and believe that they can be important to health. Some days I took 65 pills and tablets.

Now I have to consider my quality of life and must be convinced that the outcome of a therapy is worth the financial costs as well as the impact on the rest of my life. When I was getting chemotherapy, it took about 10 days out of every 30 just to recover from the chemo and get back to having MS again, which seemed like a relief. I want to hold on to the abilities that I have and to the small amount of productive time I have each day for writing, correspondence, communicating and visiting with friends, and going outside.

I have a good attitude a lot of the time and am often doing well mentally and emotionally even as I am doing quite poorly physically. Although it is terribly difficult to deal with a body that is paralyzed from the waist down and that is rapidly losing function from the waist up, I have great empathy for people suffering from things like clinical depression that I generally do not have.

I noticed some time ago that there were simply some positive improvements in my life despite the increasing MS symptoms. I noticed that I could sometimes be happy. I had previously been a busy person and somewhat of a loner. I was now a calmer person with many friends. I was moving at a much slower pace.

I feel a lot healthier in my thinking and my approach to life. Not all the time, but a lot of the fear, obsession, and worry of my previous life have fallen away. I had to be surrounded by possessions, many of which I have now given away.

Maybe one can be a healthier, calmer, more open, and patient person while having, and sometimes suffering from, a condition that is gradually robbing one of the function of the physical body. As I said to my friend Donna, it might be possible to be healed with MS even if I might not be healed from MS.

This isn't the journey that I would have chosen, and I don't know what's on the other side. I try to work on acceptance, forgiveness and appreciating what I still have. Sometimes I do not know if I can do it. I want to enjoy the good things I still have, especially my loving family and good friends. I want to learn to appreciate more fully the beauty in the world around me.

It is easy to be obsessed with what is going on with me physically. I have to remind myself that I am not alone in this. There are 300,000 people with MS in America alone. I think about those people. I know that some of them might be scared or isolated. They may not have the help and resources that I have. I also know that some of them are very accomplished and have figured out cool ways of doing things. I feel a bit competitive with those unknown people and hope that I can stack up with them.

My community has accepted and reached out to me in so many ways. I feel a responsibility to try to do this as well as I can.

I want to learn peace and patience and to love people around me. I want to learn to be there for other people even if I cannot go to their house and fix things for them. I want to learn to accept the good things that people do for me. I want to find some grace in this.

A CHEERFUL CRIPPLE

People expect me to be a cheerful cripple. After all, we all want to be around cheerful, upbeat people.

There was one evening I was less than cheerful. I had had a new $20,000 wheelchair delivered and used it for a few days. It was entirely inappropriate. It was like driving a Honda Civic around in my room. The therapist came over, and I told him it had a lot of problems. I should have been more careful because he obviously came in loaded for bear, upset about something else. I knew he was going through a rough break-up. He freaked out and screamed at me and said he would never help anyone get a wheelchair again. My sister sat there shocked and said, "What was that about?"

It took sixteen repairs and modifications to make the chair usable. I use the chair daily, and it adds immensely to my quality of life. The Arkansas Spinal Cord Commission was kind enough to help on the cost, and I paid for the rest. Handy friends did some of the work. The tilt feature switch was placed on the back of the chair where I couldn't reach it. It took two years and a lot of work for me to coordinate all the modifications, but I did it.

The therapist would not return my calls and didn't speak to me for two years and has never spoken to me about the chair or apologized.

When things go wrong, I try to be courteous. I had only been spoken to that way twice in my thirty years in business.

But after all, people do want to be around a cheerful cripple like they want to be around a cheerful person. Why would you want to visit a complaining whiner. I write my Mom every week. I had to stop calling because she complained so much about every little thing. I asked her not to complain so much. She said it's just the way she is.

I have a quadriplegic friend Pam. I have called her numerous times. She has never uttered one word of complaint. I wouldn't even know that she was in a wheelchair from speaking with her on the phone.

People just like to be around positive people. I have a great life. I have a loving spouse and a lot of amazing friends. I even have musician friends who work on concerts with me. I have a great room that Jim Key and other people remodeled to my needs. There are plenty of lonely, unhappy, disabled people. I am not one of them. I know how fortunate I am. I'm not saying it's easy, but I don't lose sight of how lucky I am.

Other people have problems of their own. Why not create a space where they can forget their problems for a while or even discuss their problems. If it's my job to be a cheerful cripple, I will accept that. There are plenty of people in the world who have it worse than I do.

WE COULD HAVE DONE ANYTHING

I went to a music camp for a number of years, and the first guy I met was named Bill Nash, and he was some kind of cripple, but I wasn't very interested in that. We camped together for three years. One year I asked him all about his condition because I was obsessed with affordable health care. He said he had something called MS. I didn't know what that was, but it seemed yucky. He was having to retire from his job and go on disability. This meant giving up his insurance which paid for his drug regimen. Just one of those drugs cost $900 per month.

I spent part of five months every year negotiating a health plan for the staff where I worked. I was committed to offering an affordable health plan to every worker. This is almost impossible. You need young people to keep your rates down, but they have different priorities. I offered a plan for $10 a month. I still couldn't recruit enough young people because $10 buys a lot of gas, beer and cigarettes. So you end up with a plan with all older workers on it.

In 2002, the young insurance guy brought me a quote of $300,000. I was flabbergasted. How the hell can any small business pay that much? I took out my pen and struck off the three oldest women and wrote in "Male, 25." The kid brought me back a very reasonable quote. This is legal discrimination. While of course I didn't really dismiss those older women, insurance companies can legally discriminate against them. Surely, many employers while they are interviewing recognize that an older woman will cost them more and pass on hiring them. Women are more likely to seek medical attention. We had lots of older women because they were great office workers with years of experience. This kind of hiring practice makes it hard to get health insurance.

We hired Della at age 60, and ten years later she celebrated her seventieth birthday on the job. She worked circles around the young kid she replaced. It was eight years before I discovered Della was a cigarette smoker. She never left her desk to take a smoke break, waiting till 5:30 so she could get to her Mustang and light up that first cigarette.

One day at music camp I saw my friend Bill sitting in the shade with his cane, and I asked him what he was up to. He said he was cooling off and getting up the energy to walk the 50 yards over to the ice cream cone booth. I asked him to let me go for him. Bill was proud and said no.

I insisted, and he finally relented. It was the most amazing walk of my life. I had never really appreciated walking until that moment. I strode freely and swung my arms and felt so free. I knew if I ever had something weird like MS, surely I would have a friend who would get ice cream for me. I never before or since felt such joy being able to walk on my own.

When I was diagnosed with MS, I called Bill. He told me he was sorry and joked that I didn't catch it from him since MS is not contagious. I didn't expect to spend long with this disease because I knew all about vitamins and health foods. Bill lives on hamburgers and beer, and his condition has progressed very little in 18 years.

Our health insurance plan at work expired every year on Woody Guthrie's birthday. I never knew if I would make the deadline. In 2002, I just made it and signed the papers, and Ginny and I left for the Woody Guthrie festival. I was obsessed with the unfairness of our health insurance system. I woke up that first morning with my head full of words about affordable health care. Ginny was understanding. She drove the 20 miles to the festival while I wrote in the car all the way. When we got there, I explained to Ginny that I had to keep writing. She was very supportive and went into the concert alone although we had had tickets for months. I wrote the song on the streets of Okemah, Oklahoma. I submitted it back to the festival. It won first place in their competition.

In 2003 they had Emily Kaitz and me open the festival with a set including this song. I was beginning to limp, and I had no idea how personal health care was about to become. People probably figured I'd had too much to drink, but Ginny was out in the audience beaming up at me, and she knew. The doctor had called before the festival and asked to speak to me, but she would not let him. He told her I had MS.

After the festival, Ginny took me out to dinner. She said, "I have something to tell you." I looked at her and said, "It's MS, isn't it?" She said, "Yes." We held hands and cried a bit. We began our new life together. I arrogantly said I would be a formidable adversary.

I realize now that Ginny and I could have done anything we put our minds to in our 30 years together. We never would have chosen a home-based MS clinic with me playing the patient. But that's what we ended up doing, with a lot of help from a lot of friends.

We could have done anything.

MS STANDS FOR MORE SO

People with MS are like everyone else except more so. MS is a metaphor for the challenges all of us face. We can hold back in fear of failure. I can't get up and speak. My voice may shake. I may have an uncontrollable urge to pee. I may fall. I may walk funny. I might not be able to get back. I might look foolish. I might be different. We have some bad days. We're not sure we can do it. But we keep trying. We choose to do some things poorly rather than not do them at all. We learn to slow down, to not be in a hurry. We laugh at our mistakes. We may cry easily. Some people claim their nerves are frayed. Ours literally are.

It is a fine line between victim and victor. We have faced one of life's greatest challenges. The average person does not know how they would respond to a debilitating condition such as MS. They may fear it. I can't blame them. We are doing it every day. We have been hit with a dreaded illness and it hasn't done us in. Yeah, we're just like everyone else. Only more so.

IT'S HIS FAULT HE'S SICK

Someone told me recently about his 90-year-old mom who is in great health because she's taking good care of herself. I was happy to hear this.

Another friend told me about her 89-year-old mother who wasn't doing well. She said, "What do you expect? She never took care of her health. She doesn't eat right." She was 89 years old. She worked all her life. Hell, maybe she got worn out taking care of you and your siblings.

I didn't just want to be healthy. I wanted to be super-healthy. I rode a bike on the weekends with my wife Ginny. I rode a bike to work in 44 minutes. I ice skated. I rollerbladed. I ate organic foods. I watched my weight. I took vitamins. I flossed.

And now I'm paralyzed and in a wheelchair.

We think if we have all the right inputs we'll get the result we want. It's a superficial understanding of karma. Ask our friends dealing with cancer. We can do everything right and sometimes life throws us a curve ball. We think we have things in order, but stuff happens.

AN EQUAL OPPORTUNITY DISEASE

MS is an equal opportunity disease. Yes, MS hits stars like Annette Funicello, Richard Pryor, Montel Williams, Terri Garr, and Squiggy from Laverne and Shirley. 200 people a week are diagnosed with MS including folks from all walks of life in our own community.

I experience becoming disabled each day. I use a wheelchair. I have lesions in the thalmic area of the brain. My problems really are all in my head. You shouldn't have to be wealthy to be disabled in this country.

Wheelchair athletes beat the runners in a marathon, is that why they make it hard to get a good wheelchair? Are they trying to keep them out of the hands of inner city wheelchair basketball players?

In any field, if you were told you had to use a certain vendor with whom there was a sweetheart contract, even though they cost more, what would you call that? Corruption? Organized crime? That is our current health insurance delivery system.

We enjoy what we have each day. If we can't walk well, we can enjoy each unique sunset. We with MS know that it is the little things that can make your day, the little kindnesses and courtesies and symbols of love and, regardless of our level of disability, we can do these things. That really is our assignment–to be the best person we can be. To have the most positive attitude we can, despite getting wacked with this severe condition, to be good to others, to be cheerful with our family if we have one, our caregivers, our friends. We really see that the little stuff that can bother folks is too little to bother with.

MS is a journey into the unknown. It is not like an injury where the patient knows their new and future status. MS changes. Some folks get better. Some get worse. Some relapse and remit. It is a life lived on the edge with no certainty. It is a life of risk. You acquire a new piece of equipment not knowing if you'll use it for ten years or ten weeks. And will it be because you are better or worse?

MS can be lonely. The struggle to deal with our disability can keep us isolated. This is not about me. I am just one of 300,000 people in this country living with MS. There are folks who are going through the same thing we are. There is someone who understands the frustrating, embarrassing, scary, unwanted problems we face each day.

INVISIBLE DISABILITIES

There's not much good about a life of disability. There are some advantages to having a very visible condition. People are more than glad to help. Look around the room. Everyone you see is dealing with significant problems in their life—all kinds of health concerns (cancer, fibromyalgia, lupus, early MS, failing eyesight), as well as finances, employment, relationships that have ended, being alone, challenges with kids. But their problems may not show. Their challenges may affect their ability to hold down a job or keep a relationship. And yet, they look perfectly normal to us.

We may wonder why the woman is using a handicap parking space and not realize that her ability to walk is limited. We may see people with problems and wonder why they don't just get over it.

But a wheelchair and a serious neurological condition tend to set you apart. People know there's really something wrong with you. But every person around us is dealing with some kind of significant challenge, and they could use our understanding and support.

LEARNING FROM CHILDREN

If I've learned anything about being a person with a disability, I've learned it from children. Children don't talk about their symptoms, the problems with getting adequate care and their changing medication regimen. It's different being around children. They just play and are interested in overcoming their disability to the point where they can participate with other children.

I love going to the Youth Center and watching the children on the climbing wall. There's the beautiful little girl with cerebral palsy who gets around with a reverse walker. She seems oblivious that she is different from the other kids. Her Mom drives up in the van and she hops in like she's done all her life. That kid is one of my role models. I talked to her one day. She nodded her chin at my chair and said, "Whatcha' got?" I said, "MS." She said, "CP. I'll see you later," and bounced back with her friends to play. I try to be like that. Maybe on my good days I get there. I know it's a blessing to be different. There are days I forget that.

Every now and then when I'm out I see the little girl with the walker and she always has a big smile on her face, not because she is overcoming some difficulty in life. She learned that a long time ago. She's just a kid who is about to have some ice cream.

It seems that children with disabilities, more so than adults, are cheerful, positive and optimistic. That's how I'd like to be. I realized that I am more than my disease, and I wanted to have some of my precious time for writing, songwriting and visiting with friends and family.

I make sure to get outside every day and to not focus on my condition, which just happens to be one of the facets of my life, a life that is rich with family and relationships with friends for which I am grateful.

If I ever got better—OK, that's highly unlikely—I would have some things to do. I'd work to be a great husband to my wife Ginny, I would try to be a comfort to the afflicted in our community, I would learn to play guitar again—I have written more than a hundred songs—and I would work with disabled children because they are my heroes.

GETTING USED TO PARALYSIS

The other morning lying in bed at about 4:30, I was cold. I knew I needed to get up and adjust the thermostat, but I was comfortable, very tired and cold. I finally awakened enough to sling my legs out of bed and go adjust the thermostat. Then I remembered, "You're paralyzed. You can't move anything." It's still hard to get used to. I've been paralyzed such a short period of my entire life. I keep thinking, "Oh, it'll go away." Instead it gets worse every single month as it has for five years. I feel like I'm in a play, and I'm just playing the part of the paralyzed guy. I try to do it as well as I can, but it doesn't seem entirely real. Fortunately, I don't have to do it alone. I've got a whole community of friends to carry me along. They make my life possible, if not easy. Thanks.

BEING ALONE VERSUS BEING LONELY

There is a difference between loneliness and being alone. I guess one difference is I know someone will be there for me–maybe in one hour, maybe two, maybe three–but there are folks that wonder if anyone will ever be there for them.

A disabled person spends a lot of time waiting–waiting for the next helper to show up, waking up and looking at the clock and seeing that you have two hours until the next helper arrives. It's not just the disabled, I realize. A lot of people have had to learn the difference between being lonely and being alone, but you certainly learn it when you're a disabled person. People set your wheelchair somewhere and say they'll be right back, and they get distracted doing something else. When people forget me, now that's lonely. I can't just go and find something to fill the time. You spend a lot of time waiting. If you're fortunate, you learn patience–deep patience. You spend the time practicing a song or a poem or maybe that essay about being alone. But you can't slip into loneliness as anyone who lives alone has learned. You find things to do or to plan or to think about. But there's a difference between being alone and being lonely.

TALK IS CHEAP

As my paralysis moves through my upper body, it affects my voice. I speak more softly and with fewer words. This works fine in my room with one other person. It doesn't work so well in a group or a crowd. People talk so fast, and they interrupt. If I do have something witty to say, by the time a space opens up, the subject has passed.

I had some version of this problem before I was disabled. I wasn't good at parties where people held a glass of wine and made small talk. I haven't had a drink in twenty-one years, and the talk was so, well, small.

I embraced song writing. I could say exactly what I wanted about a subject and reword it and rework it and eliminate excess words. I would bring my guitar to those parties, but I was too self-conscious to play my new song. At the end of the evening, I would put the guitar back in the car without ever opening the case. I could go up to a microphone in front of a room and be heard and understood, two things I really wanted.

But this isn't really communication. It is all one way. It is a shame I had to become a person with a disability to really learn to listen actively. People aren't boring. You need to know the right questions to draw them out. My friends have done cool things and been to amazing places. They are anxious to talk about these things. Now I have the time to be a good listener.

I'm still amazed at how freely people use words. People talk so loudly. They don't have the patience for my quiet response. They start a new sentence when I'm in the middle of expressing a thought. They over-explain things. They repeat themselves. They repeat themselves. They repeat the things I say. For example, if I ask for a piece of fudge, they ask me very slowly if I want a piece of fudge. They leave the room and get me something because I didn't have time to finish my sentence. Heck, words aren't cheap. They're free.

I'M NOT CRAZY, I HAVE MS

For some ten months in 2002, I began to accumulate an array of disturbing symptoms. I had coached Special Olympics for years. One night I came home from ice skating and told Ginny, "I skate like I am mentally retarded." Not that there's anything wrong with that. I loved to rollerblade for hours. Now I couldn't wait to get the skates off. I had the handwriting of a Catholic school veteran. Now I was getting brief spells where my voice would slur and my handwriting would become erratic.

Finally, in January '03, my symptoms were bad enough that I began a round of seeing countless doctors and practitioners. A 50-year-old who can't rollerskate well is hardly a neurologist's concern. Having bad handwriting is hardly a problem to a doctor. The one good piece of advice the neurologist gave me is that I should leave my stressful job. I wrote the board of directors. I told them I would stay as long as they liked. It took them four months to conduct a nationwide search. My successor, Richard, offered me the courtesy that I could stay as long as I liked, but I felt it best to get out of his way.

The highlight of that spring was the release of my CD at Mike Shirkey's, produced by Emily Kaitz. I informed all the musicians that I was having some neurological problems. They all agreed to cover for me. As it was when I felt a spell coming on, I stepped back from the mike and played a brief instrumental break. The show went off beautifully. The audience never noticed any problem.

After the show, I resumed my search for what was wrong with me. The neurologist said, "It's not like you're going to hell in a handbag." He suggested that I got psychological help. I went to a hypnotherapist. I went to a great psychologist who was the first doctor to really listen to me. He said, "I'll see you if you want, but whatever you have is not psychogenic. It's something physical." I went to a counselor. I cried that I was falling apart, and no doctor believed me.

I went to every imaginable practitioner. I finally requested, at great personal expense, a full MRI from my head to the bottom of my spine. My head was strapped down, and I was slipped into a darkened tube and told not to move, which was difficult as I had a bit of a tremor. The neurologist called Ginny and said I had MS. I had a scar or a lesion at the base of my brain in the thalmus. I had known for some time that it appeared that I had MS, but now there was a diagnosis. I excitedly called my counselor: "I'm not crazy. I have MS!" I was glad for the confirmation.

FRESHNESS

Countless people pass through my room every hour of the day and night. Friends whom I never would have known in this way. They enable me to live in my home and sleep in my own bed. They give Ginny a break. But it's more than that. I know their families and problems, and they know mine. They bring a moment of freshness in with them that I get to receive in my current vulnerable state. While I may have this condition that's left me paralyzed and in a wheelchair, I get these moments of freshness with generous people who have chosen to be a part of my life.

IT'LL MATTER

It doesn't matter how you look,
it's not important what you weigh.
It doesn't matter what you drive
or how much they're gonna pay

Don't you worry 'bout the future.
You will never change the past.
It doesn't matter if you're first,
It's no disgrace to come in last.

It doesn't matter how you move-
a limo or a chair with wheels
It's up to you that you arrive
It's up to you the way you feel.
It doesn't matter what you eat-
or else it matters quite a bit
Start askin' for advice-
you'll never hear the end of it.

But it'll matter who you touch and it matters what you give.
It'll matter if you try and makes a difference that you lived.
We're not here for very long. It's the only chance you've got.
You think it may be time to wait, but I'm thinkin' that it's not.

It doesn't matter if you're rich.
You're no less because you're poor.
It's a rolling of the dice,
not a way of keeping score.
Health and wealth are not rewards-
or used to punish if you're bad.
It's not the things you're gonna get,
or about the stuff you had.

(Song lyrics by Nick Masullo. Song included on CD *Everything You've
Got*, ASCAP@2005. Album recorded, produced, and mixed by Kelly
Mulhollan. For more information, visit www.nickmasullo.com.)

APPENDIX

COORDINATORS	CONTACT INFORMATION

POSSIBLE HELPERS	CONTACT INFORMATION

NAME OF ORGANIZATION	CONTACT INFORMATION

REGULAR HELPERS

NAME	CONTACT INFORMATION

SUBSTITUTE HELPERS

NAME	CONTACT INFORMATION

TASKS

The energy created by even a small group of people sharing a load is astounding.

TASK	TIMEFRAME	COMMENTS

ACKNOWLEDGEMENTS

The life experience that prompted this guide originates from the deep well of the community of Fayetteville, Arkansas. But the friends and family from that well extend far beyond this Ozarks community. To list every person who helped Nick and me is not possible. Another story could be told about friends, aquaintances, and total strangers who came together to raise funds and renovate our home to accommodate Nick's needs. So many people made the pain of loss *"half a sorrow."* In some small way, I hope this book returns some of that goodness.

People who put their hands into the batter of this book include women from a larger network of Fayetteville women called Ladies Lounge, women who meet monthly to discuss special topics. One month, the topic we discussed was "what would you do if faced with a debilitating illness." This discussion spawned a smaller group of women—Colleen Pancake, Nancy Varvil, Lisa Riley, Jana Stephens, and Heidi Johnston—who together conceived the idea of a simple workbook format for this book.

Additional thanks go to Rick Hinterthuer and Erika Gergerich, who offered validation that the information herein could be a valuable tool for those navigating the morass of illness.

Editor Amy Wilson at Turtle Lake Press believed in the guide and offered the needed encouragement to bring it to completion. Susan Idlet and Dot Neely volunteered their wonderful graphic design, page formatting, and editorial skills.